Top Fitness Bio-hacks

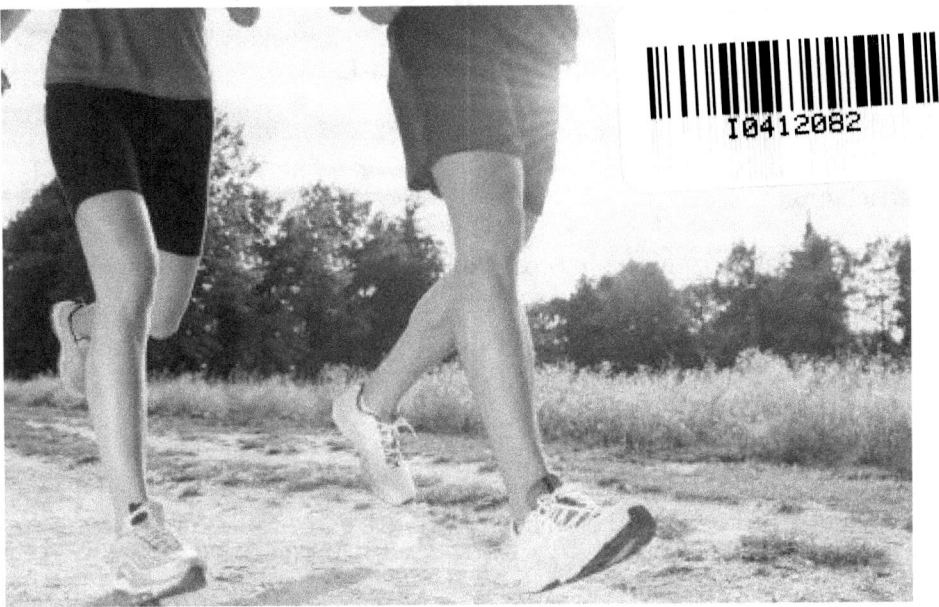

Health Learning Series

M. Usman

Mendon Cottage Books

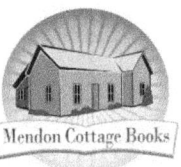

JD-Biz Publishing

Disclaimer

The information is this book is provided for informational purposes only. It is not intended to be used and medical advice or a substitute for proper medical treatment by a qualified health care provider. The information is believed to be accurate as presented based on research by the author.

The contents have not been evaluated by the U.S. Food and Drug Administration or any other Government or Health Organization and the contents in this book are not to be used to treat cure or prevent disease.

The author or publisher is not responsible for the use or safety of any diet, procedure or treatment mentioned in this book. The author or publisher is not responsible for errors or omissions that may exist.

Warning

The Book is for informational purposes only and before taking on any diet, treatment or medical procedure, it is recommended to consult with your primary health care provider.

Our books are available at
1. Amazon.com
2. Barnes and Noble
3. Itunes
4. Kobo
5. Smashwords
6. Google Play Books

Table of Contents

Prelude

Biohacking is the science, or more specifically an art, that is based upon the hacker ethic whose aim is to maximize the potentials of your body so you can live a longer, healthier life. The whole concept if biohacking lies on the foundations of do-it-yourself so you won't be able to gain success until and unless you are willing to engage your body in self-experimentation. With respect to fitness, biohacks are a tad bit complex, in a sense that they would be pretty much personal to everyone and one generic hack would hardly apply to each individual. A little deeper and it would mean that biohacks would depend on the topic of interest, which could either be increased power, muscle, or fitness. The whole methodology of biohacks is threefold, which is explained in the subsequent paragraphs.

If you're really on a quest for better, healthier lifestyle, the foremost thing that you need to have evaluated is yourself. A number of people are wizards in pointing out all things one shouldn't do but fail to list all the things they should do. The best way to do so is by tracking your progress and noting every worthwhile detail like sleeping patterns, exercise plans, etc.

The next thing you should consider is change. Change is vital for life in a sense that it must keep some excitement in life. You must be able to tweak the details and routines of your life. Change your diet plan, sleeping patterns, an anything else that makes you more comfortable. If you can track it, you can change it.

What might work for one person might not work for you; you have to realize this much. You need to know that not every person has the same physical and chemical characteristics as the other and to achieve optimal health you must have an open mind that could induce flexibility in your thinking.

The last three paragraphs are the basic ground rules that should be in your mind if you plan on transforming your health into something worth showing off. The exact techniques to do this have been explained in the book, so read on.

Identifying Fitness

Most of use the word fitness in our lives as if it means nothing, but being a little more specific, what are the factors that decide the level of fitness a person has? Fitness, specifically talking about physical fitness, is a collection of attributes that must be attained by a person in order to efficiently perform everyday tasks. Fitness is something that is dependent on perspective; what might be healthy and justified for some might be too little for you or vice versa. This diversity can create a little problem in specifically defining fitness, but still scientists have been able to come up with a few parameters that can correctly define fitness:

i.   Cardiopulmonary functions:

The body is fed fuel in the form of glucose and oxygen which is used in each and every function in the body, all the way down to blinking. This implicitly means that your physical fitness is directly dependent on the efficiency of the cardiopulmonary system and its characteristics.

ii.   Body composition:

To attain tip top physical fitness, it is absolutely necessary that the body be of the perfect height as well as weight. A quantity known as BMI is the perfect marker for body composition, which is used in several departments for classifying obesity of an individual. A Body Mass Index in between 20 and 25 is ideal and looking over at either side of the spectrum you would either be too thin or too obese. In the same way, another characteristic that could judge a person's body composition is fat percentage of the body. It is necessary to understand that there is a limit to the amount of fat the body can have. Any higher than that and the body could suffer:

- For women, lower limit 5%, upper limit 35%.

- For men, lower limit 5%, upper limit 25%

iii.   Muscle Strength:

The definition of muscle strength is the extent of force the muscles can exert while doing a physical task. The difference between a normal individual and a weight lifter is that of muscle strength; explosive strength is made available to the body through the action of twitch muscle fibers. More will be discussed later.

iv.   Endurance:

Endurance is synonymous with stamina. It means that this is the amount of physical activity a person can carry out without tiring. It's an important factor that decides the fitness and well-being of a person. The slow twitch muscles in your muscles define your endurance and those are the ones that should be focused on in order to improve endurance.

Bio-hacking

Chapter # 1: Nutrition, Exercise & Sleep

Fitness is not something that only athletes and sportsman can and/or should strive to achieve. A common person is as much eligible to optimum fitness as any other professional. The three most basics steps to fitness for a commoner are nutrition, exercise, and sleep, all of which will be explained in the chapter.

Nutrition:

What you eat and how you eat it defines the level of wellness you can obtain from an edible item. The book will support the traditional statement of breakfast being the most vital meal of the day, primarily because the brain needs a lot of energy to perform the basics tasks of the day at work or at school. The brain needs glucose, but there is an alternative as well: ketone bodies. Ketone bodies are a great substitute for the sugary and fatty ingredients in your breakfast. For instance, substituting a tablespoon of butter with coconut oil would provide you with all the energy you need.

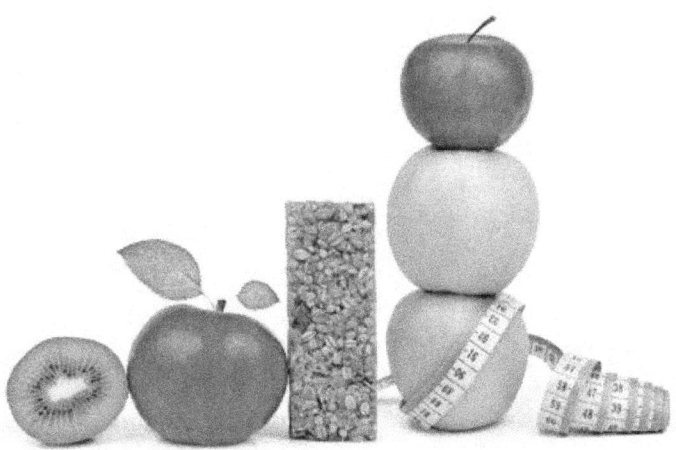

For lunch, dinner, and snacks, the best product to eat is red or white meat which comes from pasture-fed animals. Whole products are a lot more nutritious than processed ones. At the same time it must be understood that it is not entirely appropriate to drop all the meat and stick to vegetables only as meats are a great source of much needed antioxidants, minerals, vitamins and fatty acids.

How you eat it can also have an influence over your physical fitness. The theory of having something in your mouth all day long is wrong and in fact researchers are proving time and again that intermittent eating patterns can be much healthier. A particular eating plan that could do you a lot of good is known as intermittent fasting, which requires you to fast at particular times. The method will provide you with guaranteed results.

Exercise:

Some people feel tired after a workout instead of active; they feel like the results are taking too long and view the whole routine as something that slows them down. If you're one of these people then maybe you need to rethink your whole strategy. The first thing you need to do is replace your routine with whole body vibration regimens. Most of the professional athletes have already shifted to this technique and results of a Greek study have shown that subjects who underwent 6 week sessions of WBV experienced an increase in strength, stamina, and power.

Mood:

No matter what your physical fitness is, as long as you are screaming from the inside, you won't do yourself any good. A bitter mood is not only responsible for taking away serenity, but also causes hormonal imbalance which leads to many disorders. You must have heard about the benefits of breathing exercises in controlling anxiety, depression, and etc. This book will tell you how you can bio-hack your way to an enlightened mood. A technique known as heart rate variability biofeedback can help synchronize heart beat and bring back focus to your life. Studies have shown that this method can sometimes prove more superior to yoga and can bring calm to baroreceptors, while lowering the amount of stress hormones.

Sleep:

This is one of the most underrated aspects of a healthy life, even though people spend a large part of their lives sleeping. Newer research has shown that the quantity of sleep a person gets is not dependent on the level of comfort or relaxation obtained. In fact, the quality of sleep is much more important and humans can carry out daily tasks quite comfortably with just a few hours of sleep every day. Sleeping in a dark room with the right type of diet and getting up right on time are all necessary factors for better health.

Chapter # 2: Muscle Growth

If you're looking to improve your muscle mass, then the typical technique of looking after your reps won't get you anywhere. There are specialized methods that can help you build more muscle:

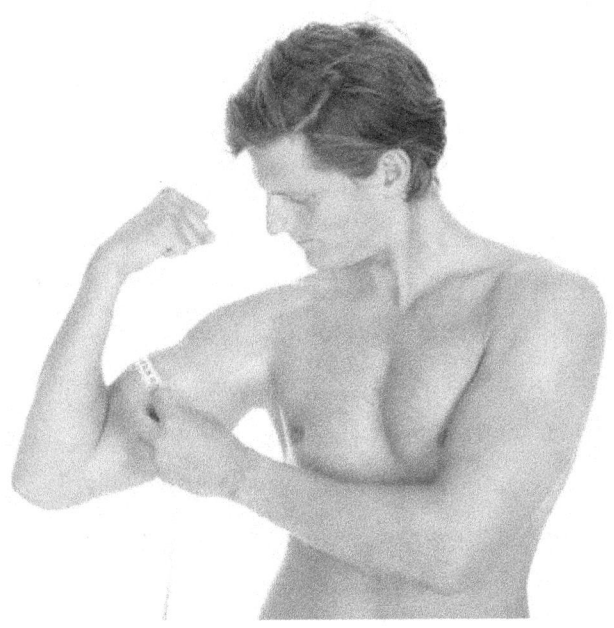

➤ **Time under Tension:**

When it comes to increasing muscle, the first priority should be following the right technique. This is where a TUT regimen comes in. This regimen involves putting the muscles under strain for as long as possible, so that they can gain maximum endurance and with that, maximum muscle. There is no doubt that reps matter, but if you're thinking of sacrificing quality then the results won't be those that are expected.

This particular training method is much more superior to other workouts mainly because it keeps in mind the biological factors of the body. The body is set to adopt the conditions it is put in. When a muscle fiber is stretched for a long enough time it increases in length. This process is known as hypertrophy and is exactly what this method succeeds in achieving.

> **Workout supplements:**

The right type of supplements can give you a guaranteed edge in your objective of obtaining increased muscle mass.

i.   BCAA:

BCCAs or branched chain amino acids are one of the most taken supplements among athletes and builders. They greatly enhance muscle activities after workouts and decrease the intensity of breakdown in muscles, which gives them such a high place among individuals. Studies have supported this statement and have repeatedly proven that BCAAs are more efficient than other supplements. Moreover, the major source of energy is glycogen which is found right in the muscles. BCAAs are responsible for making sure that they don't run out too quickly and last long enough for enduring tasks.

ii.   Beta Alanine:

This supplement might not be directly responsible for increasing muscle mass, but it does have effects that indirectly result in it. The major limitations that an individual faces while performing any kind of workout is fatigue, which leads to tiredness, and that ultimately reduces the duration and intensity of workout. Research has shown that an increase in the muscle's acidity or pH can result in increased amount of fatigue. Therefore it is only reasonable that the level of acidity be countered. This can be accomplished using a chemical called carnosine which is formed through the synthesis of beta-alanine. Once the carnosine in the muscles has neutralized the acidic chemicals, the body is once again ready to work at full pace.

iii.   Carbohydrates:

Carbohydrates should not be forgotten as an ingredient to greater muscles. Carbohydrates are vital for improving the status of proteins during workouts through two mechanisms. The first one involves the use of carbohydrates in exercises of lighter intensities, whereas in the longer run, carbohydrates make sure that the body's glycogen reserves do not run out, which enables the body to engage in exercises for much longer.

Chapter # 3: Fat Loss

Fat loss is not only responsible for making you more attractive physically, but also helps the body get rid of many diseases like diabetes, obesity, etc. The following techniques can be applied to counter obesity:

➢   **Weight training vs. Aerobics:**

Ask any gym goer for the method he/she uses to burn fat and to gain muscles. Their reply will be similar to the reply of thousands of others: cardio for fat loss and weight-training for muscles. But, one needs to question themselves if that method is truly effective.

The type of exercise a person chooses largely describes the individual's physical desire. Some people tend to prefer aerobics, while some go with lifting weights. But keeping in mind your goal of fat loss, you might want to have a varied preference. It is a well-established statement that aerobics can significantly reduce fat content in our bodies, while weight training can only help with protein gains.

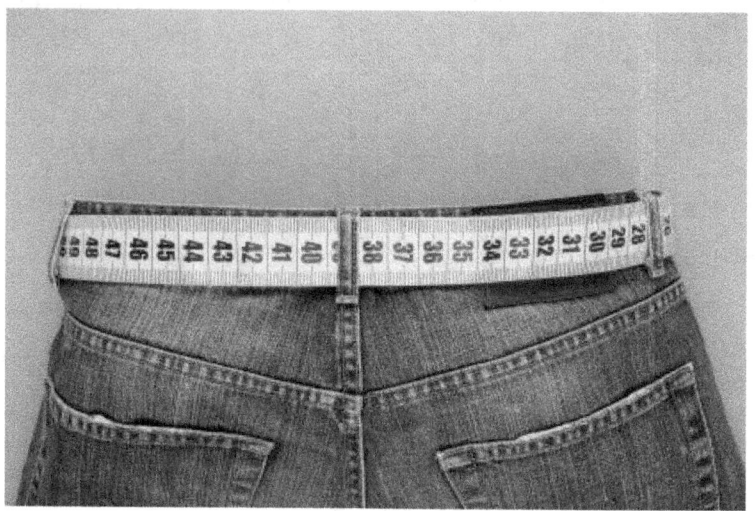

Just like resistance and high intensity interval training, weight training is proving to be a better alternative to fat-loss regimens; newer research is proving this. Weight training is able to greatly increase the post-exercise oxygen intake which shows that the body is working at a higher metabolic rate than before. A higher metabolic rate automatically translates to greater fat loss. Moreover, another research claims that the benefits of aerobic exercises with respect to fat loss are negligible which greatly highlights the need to shift towards weight training.

However, exercises like HIIT still show significant progress with respect to fat loss as it increases oxidation of fat through different mechanisms. One major mechanism through which it accomplishes fat loss is through increasing the oxidation of fat enzymes in the skeletal muscle structure. HIIT, in combination with other types of weight training, can also cause increased muscle mass which means an increase in the basal metabolic rate. An increase in metabolic rate means increased fat oxidation! Also, aerobics are not very popular when it comes to increasing the testosterone level. On the other hand, HIIT and RT are very good at it, which in turn causes an increase in the pace of fat loss. Last but not the least, you get more benefits by spending lesser time in weight training than aerobics, so why sideline such a beautiful technique.

> ## Keeping Maximal Oxygen Uptake in the Burning Zone:

If still, after all reasoning, you wish to go towards aerobics, there are a few suggestions for you that can ensure better performance. The foremost one is keeping your oxygen uptake in the fat burning area. What is this strange area? Studies have shown that individuals who go through aerobic exercises can lose more weight when they are performing at 70% heart rate.

> ## Cold Thermogenesis:

Another very productive method for training is cold thermogenesis. Compared to rigorous morning workouts, it is a much better method and can greatly assist a person with fat loss. The first thing required for this is splashing cold water over ones face or sitting in an ice bath for some time. The idea might sound strange for a minute, but actually it is very efficient. Whenever you feel cold, the body starts to vibrate or shiver in order to generate heat. This heat is generated from body fat and therefore cold thermogenesis involves cooling down the body to a level that it uses body fat to start itself up. Fat loss is not the only benefit of thermogenesis:

i.   Ice or cold water prevents joints from swelling after exercise.

ii.   The colder body temperature also shuts down activation of muscle spindles which relieves pain.

Explosive power exercises are performed with the goal of creating more force in less amount of time. Every athlete strives to achieve this goal which is by training in an explosive manner: lifting heavy weights in shorter time intervals:

Explosive Power Drills:

These exercises shouldn't be performed in an individual manner, but must be a part of a training routine.

i. **Plate jump** – This exercise features the weights in a forceful forward swing. The forward swing has a resulting forward pull on the body which forces the body to equalize the speed of the weights to prevent a fall in the forward direction. On each rep, a person should try to jump as fast and hard as possible and should reset his/her stance after each jump. The possible variations that can be brought in this exercise include height, distance, and weight.

To perform this exercise, get hold of a 10 pound plate in each hand and stand straight. While keeping the body in a downward position, swing the plate in a backwards direction. Next, as you jump, swing the plate upward and forward simultaneously and let the weights carry you as you do so. Perform 3 sets of 8 reps of this exercise.

ii. **Frog squat jump** – The principle behind this exercise is switching to full force in a fast and concentric manner. The resulting contractions cause an increase in force in a lesser amount of time.

To perform this exercise, hold the end of a dumbbell using both hands and stand straight. Keep the free end of the dumbbell in a downwards direction and relax your arms. Keeping this pose, jump forward and while jumping, keep your arms straight; perform 3 sets of 8 reps each.

iii. **Kettle Bell Quick Step** – This exercise is the first step for individuals training to be fighters. It improves their punching and kicking power.

In order to perform this exercise, initiate a normal swing before taking a big step in the forward direction using one leg. Drive in the forward direction with the other leg whole the bell ascends and as soon as the kettle bell reaches the chest level, move the leg in a forward direction.

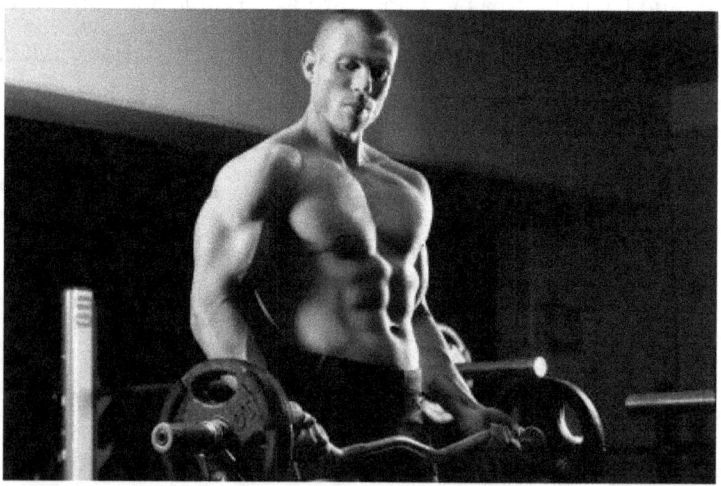

iv. **Jumping lunges** – These movements are very beneficial for athletes who require leg movements to get warmed up.

To perform this exercise, assume lunge position making sure that the toes are in line with the chest. Extend your legs and start switching your legs in mid-air while moving in the forward direction. Use your arms to maintain balance and perform 3 sets of 6 reps.

v. **Bulgarian Jump Squat** – This is one of the most tedious exercises in this book, but is equally effective in developing explosive power.

In order to execute this exercise, rest one of the legs on the bench and other one right on the floor. Develop enough power in the knee of the back leg so that it lifts from the ground. Swing the arms as if you are about to sprint on one leg which would maximize your balance; the recommended reps are 8 with 3 sets.

vi. **Dumbbell Swing Three Jump** – This exercise may also be called a combination of pull-through and dumbbell swings. Instead of using arms as a base for initiating jumping, the hips are used.

To perform this exercise, hold the end of a dumbbell using both the hands. The free end of the dumbbell should always be facing the forward direction. Drop you head now so that the dumbbell swings between the legs and attempt to reach as far as possible. Move the hips forward and jump which would allow you to speed up the dumbbell. A large amount of force would be created as a result of the movement, which will allow you to perform this exercise; the recommended set number is 3 with 6 reps each.

Chapter # 5: Increased Strength

Building muscles that look massive in appearance is not just the desire of bodybuilders, but also of regular gym members. Additional bulk may be the requirement of many physical activities, but it is definitely not a necessity; strength, on the other hand, is a necessity. There are numerous performers, boxers, and fighters who increase their strength on a regular basis without ever putting on extra weight. Strength is not really a property of muscles, but of the motor system.

Weight training is a technique that not only adds bulk to the body but also increases strength. One thing that must be understood is that there is a hefty amount of difference between the techniques and required results of power lifters and body builders. Power lifters are those athletes who work for increasing raw strength in their bodies; they don't focus on adding bulk and use heavier weights throughout their regimens. On the other hand, bodybuilders go for muscle size increase and apply all methods that would make them bulkier.

Whenever a person exercises his/her skeletal muscles increase in size in a process known as hypertrophy. There are two major directions which the body can take in order to increase bulk size of muscles. The first one involves real increase in the elements of skeletal muscles and the structures that form the muscle fibers are paralleled so that there is an increase in the muscle strength and size. The second type of hypertrophy, which is known as "sarcoplasmic hypertrophy", comes as a result of increase in muscle size in conjunction with an increase in non-contractile entities. This type of hypertrophy involves accumulation of connective tissues, fats, etc. which results in an increase in muscle size; however there is little increase in function of the muscles.

Similarly, the two types of lifting, namely powerlifting and bodybuilding, focus on two different mechanisms of hypertrophy. Bodybuilders and athletes who aim to build bulk should focus on lifting lesser weights, but more sets and reps, which would prevent muscles from reaching maximum stretching. These conditions induce sarcoplasmic hypertrophy which is exactly what a bodybuilder needs. At the same time, you must be made aware of the analogy that this particular type of hypertrophy is more or less something similar to pumping fluid into your muscle. This means that the muscles will only get bigger but not stronger. This is exactly why bodybuilders look good only in pictures, but fail in strength tasks versus much thinner individuals.

Power lifters however are concerned lesser about their appearance and more about their real power. The type of hypertrophy these guys use is the one that comes from increasing the size of contractile muscles in the skeletal units. The lifters need to be focused on performing lesser reps but with heavier weights. The optimum output is obtained when the muscles are pushed to the limit. When the muscles undergo maximum stretching, they would require more myofibrils to match up with the required performance which results in hypertrophy or an increase in muscle size. The strength achieved through this mechanism is unmatched.

Factors Affecting Endurance

Endurance training is something that always brings cardio to our minds whenever it is pronounced. There is no doubt about the statement that cardio has a significant role in endurance training, but that is not the end of it. Strength training is also a part of endurance training as it also has the same objectives as those put out for cardio based exercises. A very important parameter which would judge an athlete's performance is maximal oxygen uptake or VO2 max, which in simple words, is the maximum rate of oxygen consumed throughout the workout. Oxygen, as you know it, is a basic fuel that is required to produce energy and if the body gets a sufficient amount of the fuel, it can provide energy to the muscles smoothly. This factor or parameter is controlled by the cardiovascular system. Most endurance athletes therefore train their cardiovascular system, which results in a better control over VO2 max.

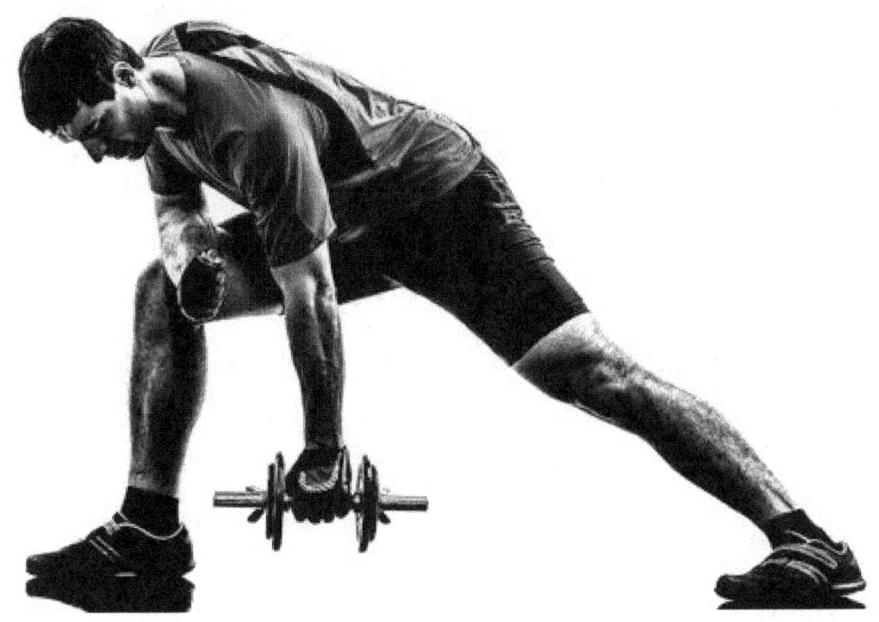

Better maximal oxygen uptake can be achieved using a few tips and tricks in your workout. The following are a few ways:

1.   Strength exercises:

The muscles and cardiopulmonary system need to become stronger and to do that, more and more muscle fibers should participate in physical activities. The best way to do this is by combining the cardio with strength days. Many people usually allocate different days for the two different types of exercises but the best way to maximize benefits is by combining both. For instance, combine bench press with pushups followed by a 4 – 6 minute long run.

2.   Dynamic warm-up:

Warm ups are a key part of exercise, but most people tend to overlook it and switch directly to high intensity exercises. This only ruins an individual's workout by failing the body of oxygen. A research carried out by Ohio University showed that a proper warm up can help achieve over 25% of the maximal oxygen uptake, but no warm up results in a slower increase in the uptake.

3.   Quality:

Quality over quantity; make this a rule of life. People think that they will be able to build their strength or add bulk to their bodies simply by increasing the number of executions of a particular exercise. But in reality, quality has a definite edge over quantity. The quality of a workout means that whatever routine you buildup for yourself, you must follow it. Moreover, you should be near perfect in your posture and execution, or else you would be working out the wrong muscle.

4.   Staying hydrated:

For almost every endurance exercise, staying hydrated is the perfect strategy. Talking in general, being un-hydrated for a significant amount of time can result in the initiation of electrolyte depletion, which can soon affect cognitive abilities. Moreover, the drop in electrolytes also causes cramps and fatigue. Thus, any person, professional or amateur, should make sure that he/she consumes at least 16 – 24 ounces of water before a workout. ½ of your body mass in ounces is recommended for athletes who go on strenuous, sweating workouts. For example, say you weigh 170 pounds; this means that you should be gulping 85 ounces of water a day.

5.   Popular endurance exercises:

Different endurance exercises exist for athletes which include swimming, jogging, cycling, dancing, climbing hills, basketball, etc.

6.   Proteins:

A balanced diet is essential for a rewarding workout and what rewards a person more than a powerhouse class of compounds known as protein. Proteins contain amino acids which are essential for the body's growth. You are advised to consume at least 1 gram of protein for every kilo gram of your body weight on a daily basis.

7.   Carbohydrates:

During workouts, a lot of energy is lost and glycogen reserves are emptied. As a compensation for this waste, the diet should contain plenty of carbohydrates which would replenish the whole supply. Carbohydrates may be used either during or after workouts to enhance workout output. About 2 – 3 grams of carbohydrates a day for every kilogram of body weight is recommended to all those concerned about their health. The different sources of carbohydrates include vegetables, fruits, oatmeal, etc.

8.   Supplements:

Moreover, it is also very healthy for you to add supplements to your diet; supplements which actively improve endurance include:

a.   Energy boosting beverages.

b.   Stimulant products.

9.   Relaxation:

Rest before, during, and after workouts is as important as the workout itself. Most people tend to rest for a minute while many feel replenished in just half a minute. Endurance workouts are designed so that rest times can be minimized. Experts suggest that the muscles should be put under so much stress that it totally gives up. Only then can the workout stop. Rest should be used as a measure to prevent injury otherwise the workout should go on. 10 reps of each of the following exercise would provide you with a good idea of endurance routines: squats, pull-ups, pushups, and jogging. Each of the exercises should have a minimal amount of break between them.

10.   Interval training:

What is meant by interval training? Interval training is basically a workout routine which shifts between low intensity and high intensity routines at separate intervals. For instance, if a person decides to jog for 15 minutes, he/she should probably run at a normal pace during the first 5 minutes of the jog then the person should gradually increase his speed during the next 5 minutes and during the last 5 minutes the person should start brisk walking. Studies have clearly shown that when interval training is used, the rate of increase in maximal oxygen uptake increases dramatically and the chances of injury are also reduced.

11.   Training at Altitude:

High altitude training has also been found to have a positive effect on the maximal oxygen uptake of individuals. Many physiological changes occur in a person's body when he/she trains at higher altitude; the function of heart and respiratory system dramatically increases. This change can be observed from the heavy breathing that a person encounters at high altitudes. This heavy breathing results in a change in the acid-base balance of the body which ultimately leads to an increase in the maximal oxygen uptake. Despite lower oxygen concentration, the body is still able to reap the benefits of high altitude through a process known as "erythropoiesis". When the body is exposed to a lower concentration of oxygen in the atmosphere, there is a similar interest on the body concentration of oxygen which also decreases. This decrease has a direct effect on the kidneys, which detect the change and start production of a chemical known as erythropoietin. This hormone is basically a signal for increasing the number of red blood cells by sending a message to the bone marrow. Once the concentration of the cells increases, more oxygen is carried, at lower oxygen levels. This explains the fact as to why people who dwell in regions of high altitude never face a problem in breathing in low oxygen conditions.

But at the same time, it must also be stated that no exercise is best at high altitude and one must keep experimenting till he/she hits the right combination.

Another way of reaping the benefits of high altitude is by working out in a CVAC, which is a pod with variable air parameters. It functions essentially as a high altitude environment, but is still not in widespread use due to lack of blind trust from medical researchers and practitioners.

Conclusion

At the end of it all, everything boils down to genetics. Like all other aspects of the human body and its performances, genetics have the last say in every matter. No matter how much you train, if your genes don't have a particular quality in them, you won't develop it. Over 200 genes in the body control different physical parameters. However, the book has very elaborately described hacks to fitness in the most suitable way which can now be used by anyone to make his/her life better. An intermediate biohacker may find this book very useful since it uses concepts like maximal oxygen uptake and endurance parameters. But, still the concepts are very basic and any enthusiast, which is basically what a biohacker is, should be able to understand it. Best of luck practically applying it!

Author Bio

Muhammad Usman is a distinguished medical graduate of Allama Iqbal medical college (AIMC). He is a professional writer who has been in the field for more than 4 years. During this time he has produced 10,000+ articles, blogs and eBooks on various niches related to diseases, health, fitness, nutrition and well-being. He is a regular contributor to several journals related to medicine and surgery. He is the editor of several journals and newspapers.

References

http://www.123rf.com/photo_22583738_legs-view-of-a-couple-jogging-outdoor-in-the-park.html

http://www.123rf.com/photo_20519460_one-caucasian-man-exercising-weight-training--on-white-background.html

http://www.123rf.com/photo_15701414_chocolate-muesli-bars-with-apple-and-kiwi-isolated-on-white-background.html?term=nutrition

http://www.123rf.com/photo_23934531_man-measuring-his-biceps-with-measuring-tape-on-white-background.html?term=muscle%20growth

http://www.123rf.com/photo_21428477_jeans-with-meter-belt-slimming-on-the-green-background.html?term=fat%20loss

http://www.123rf.com/photo_22087941_strong-man--bodybuilder-with-dumbbells-in-a-gym-exercising-with-a-barbell.html?term=strength

Check out some of the other JD-Biz Publishing books

Gardening Series on Amazon

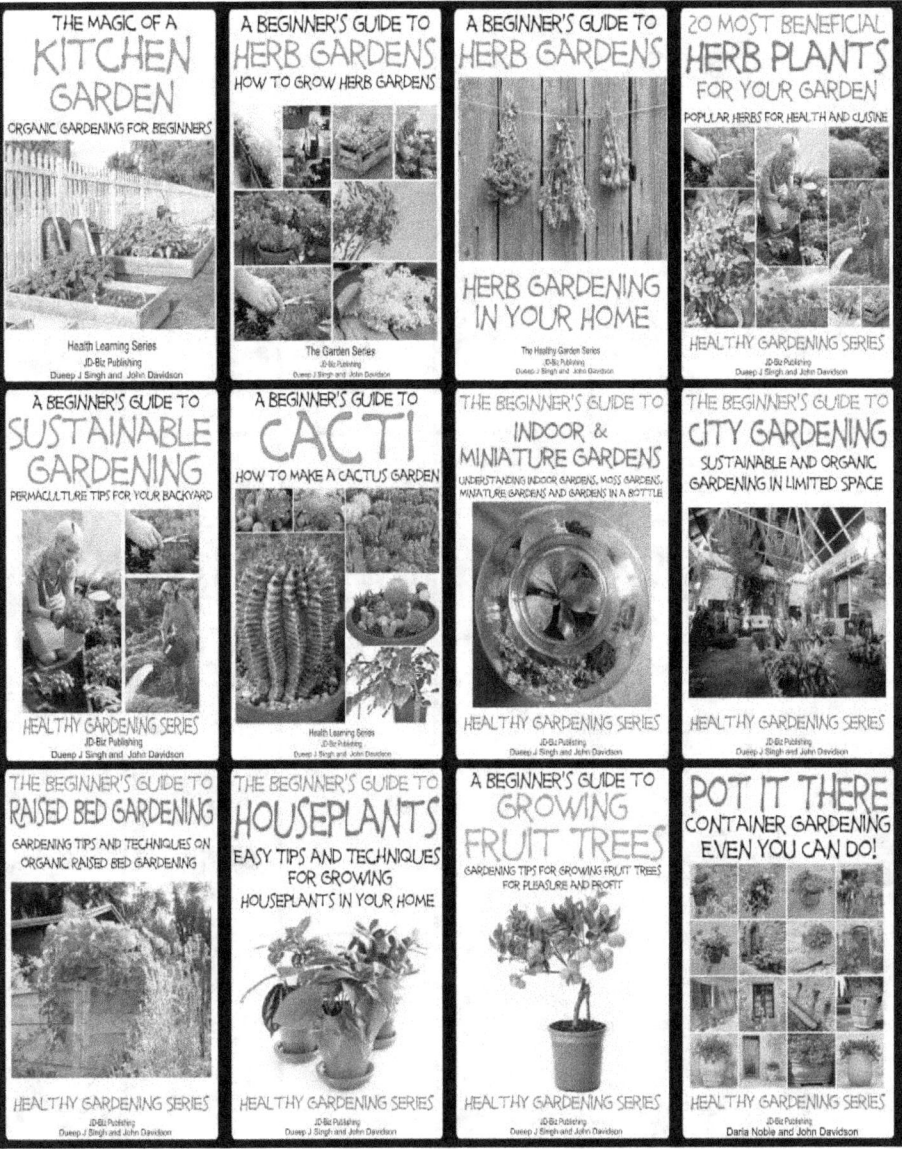

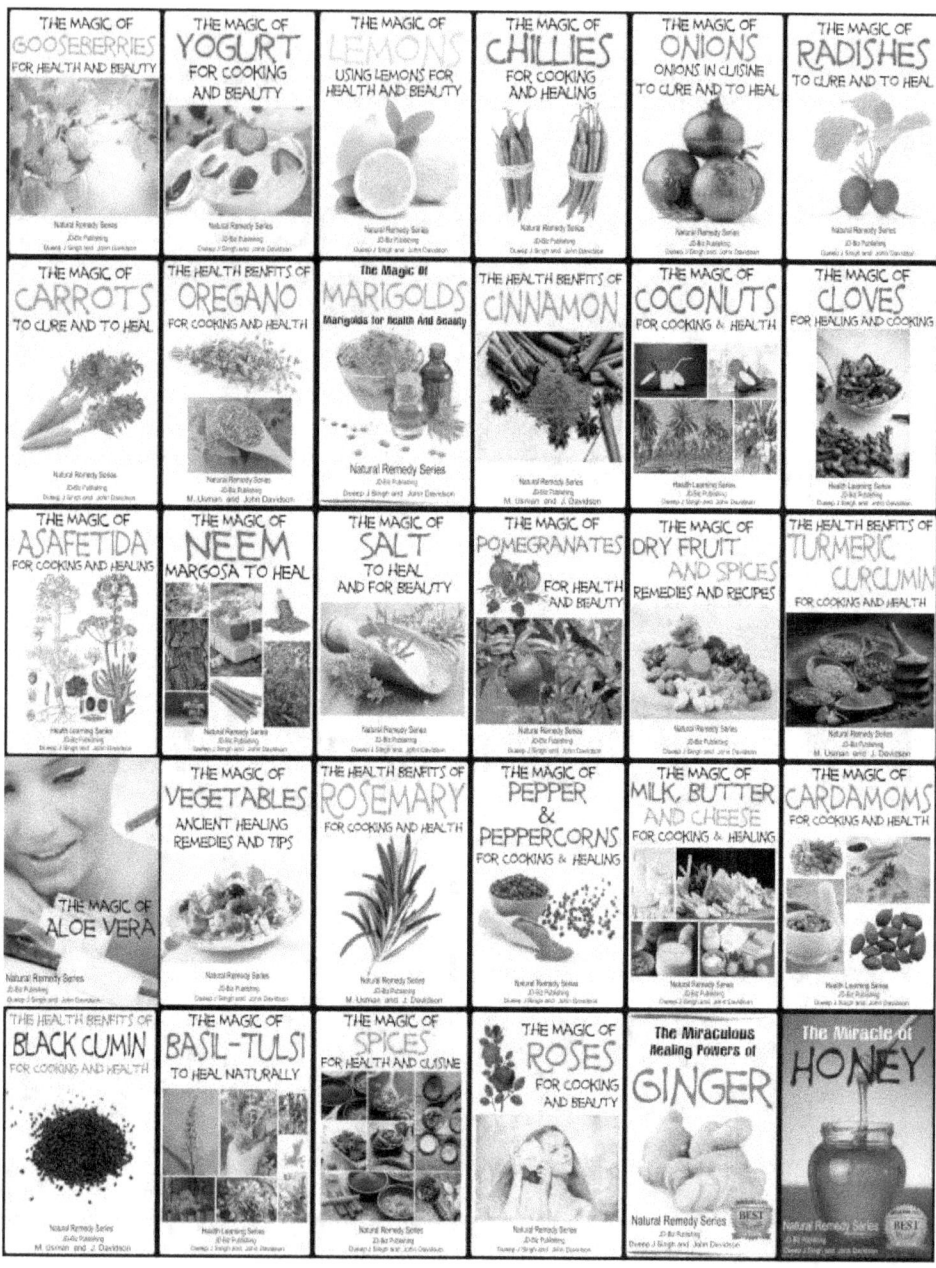

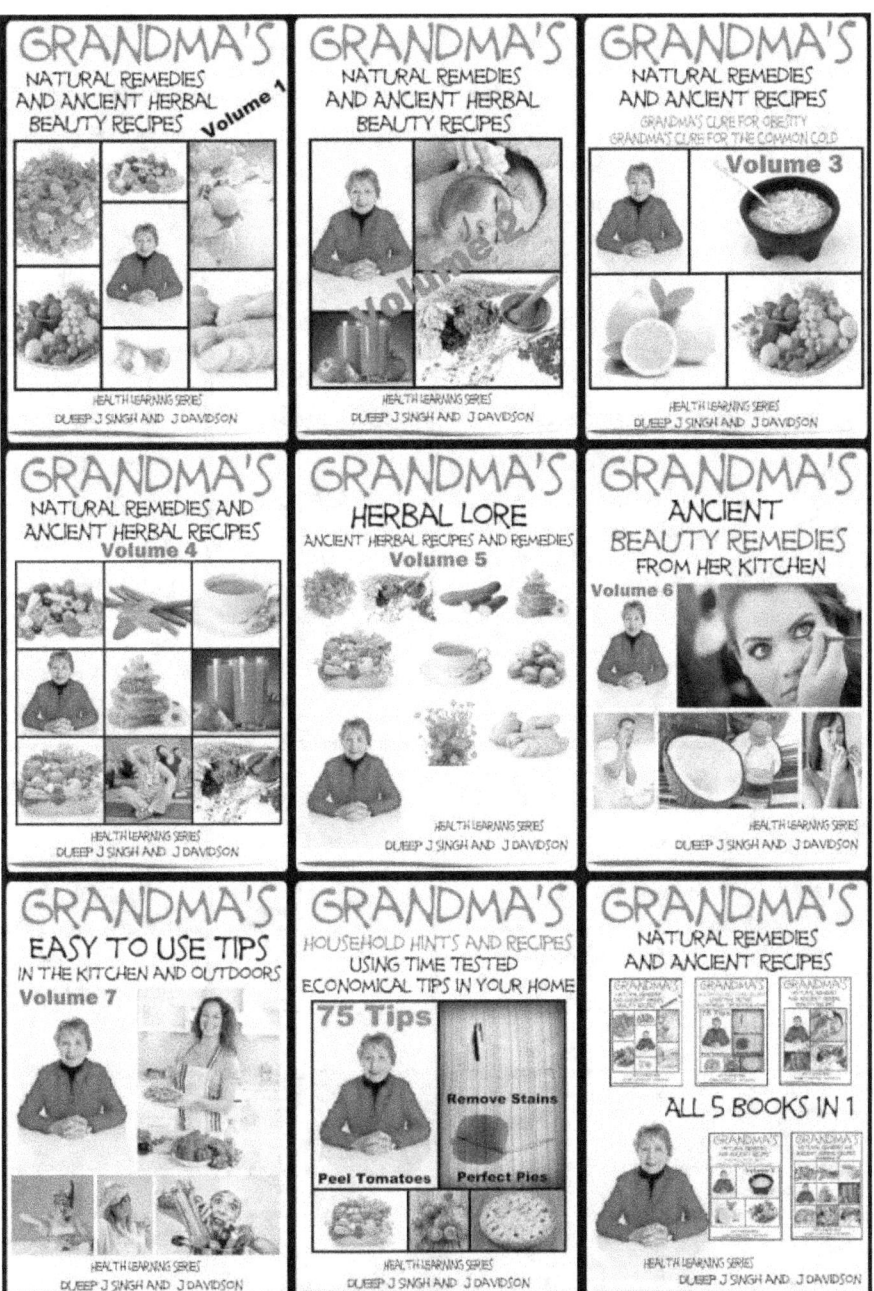

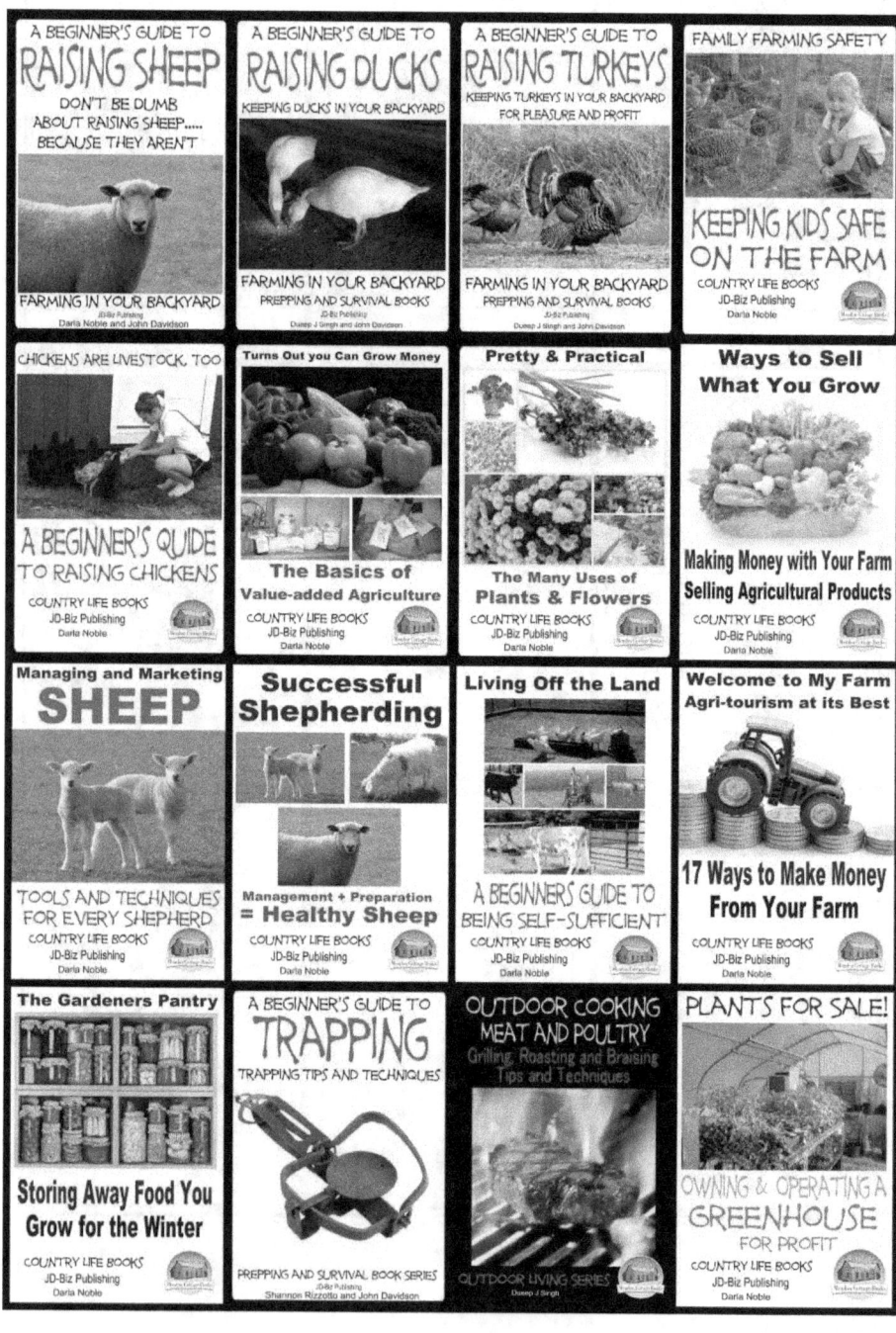

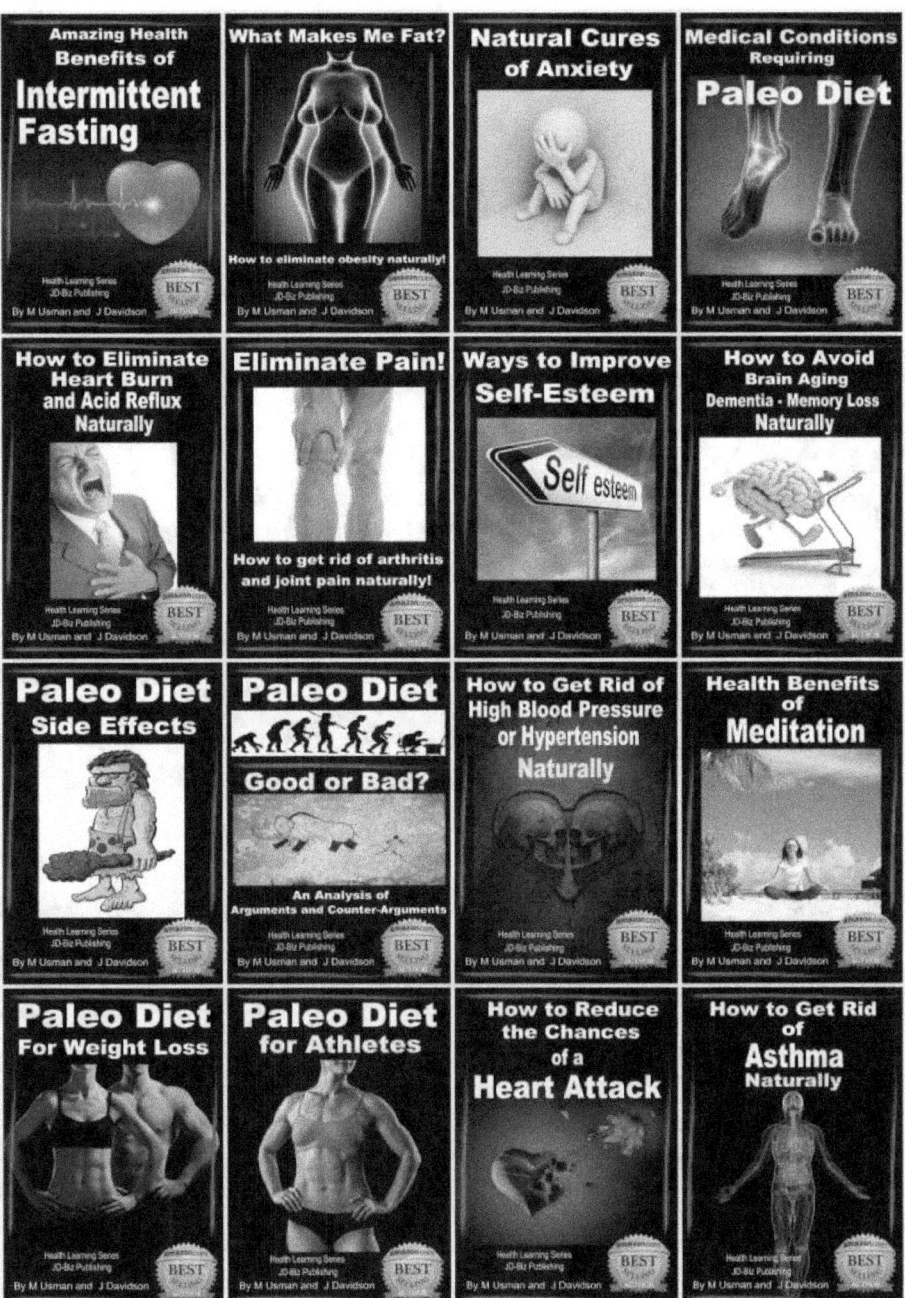

<u>Amazing Animal Book Series</u>

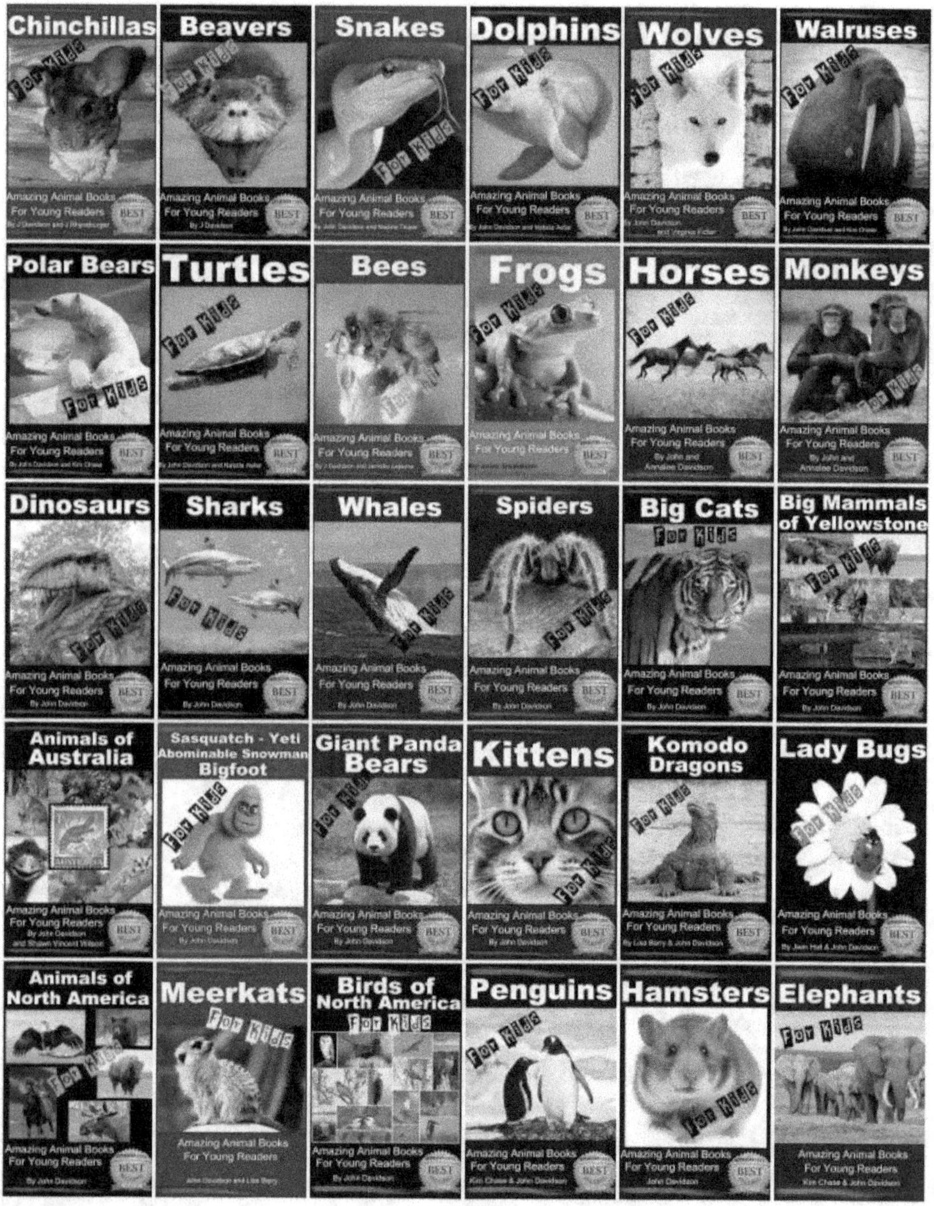

Learn To Draw Series

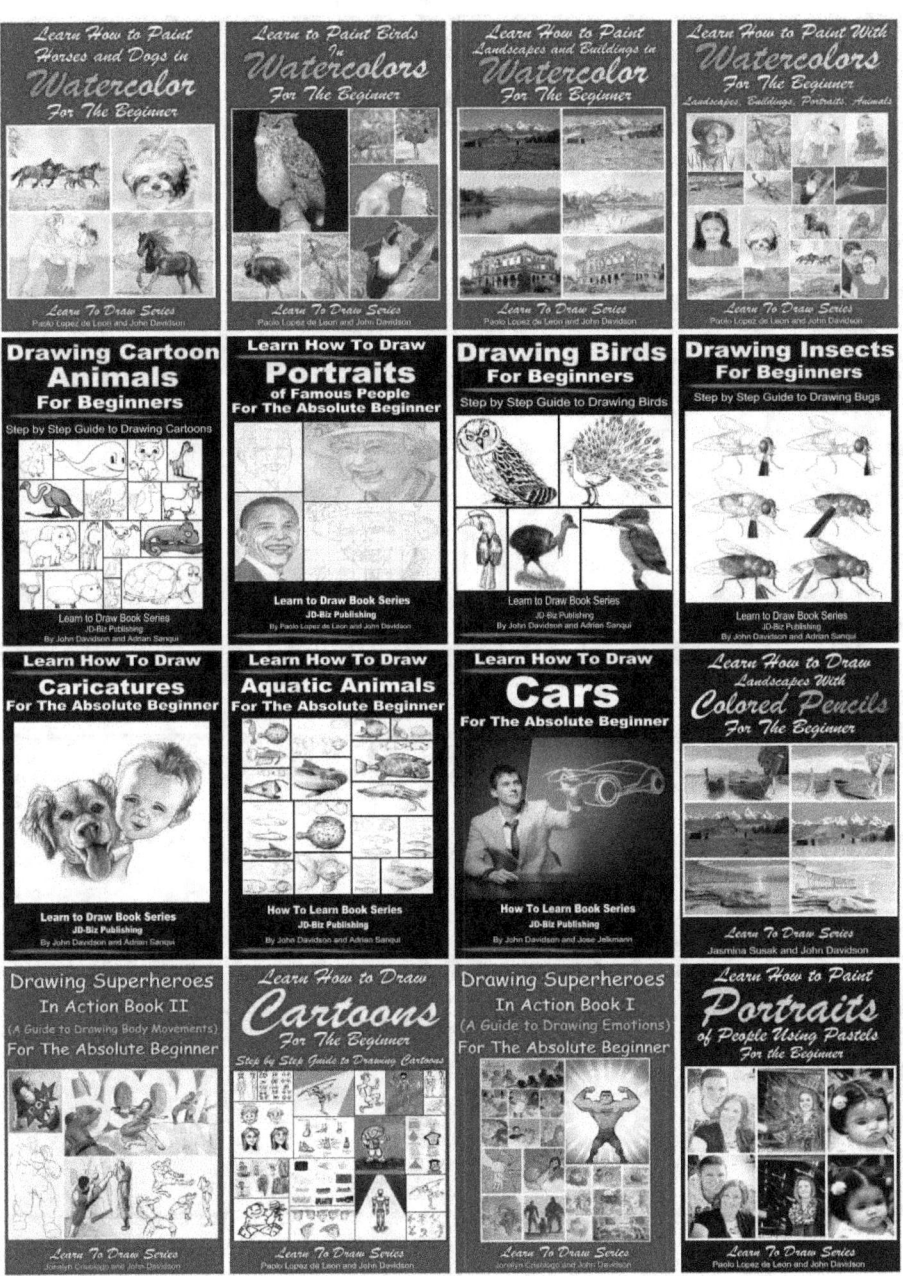

How to Build and Plan Books

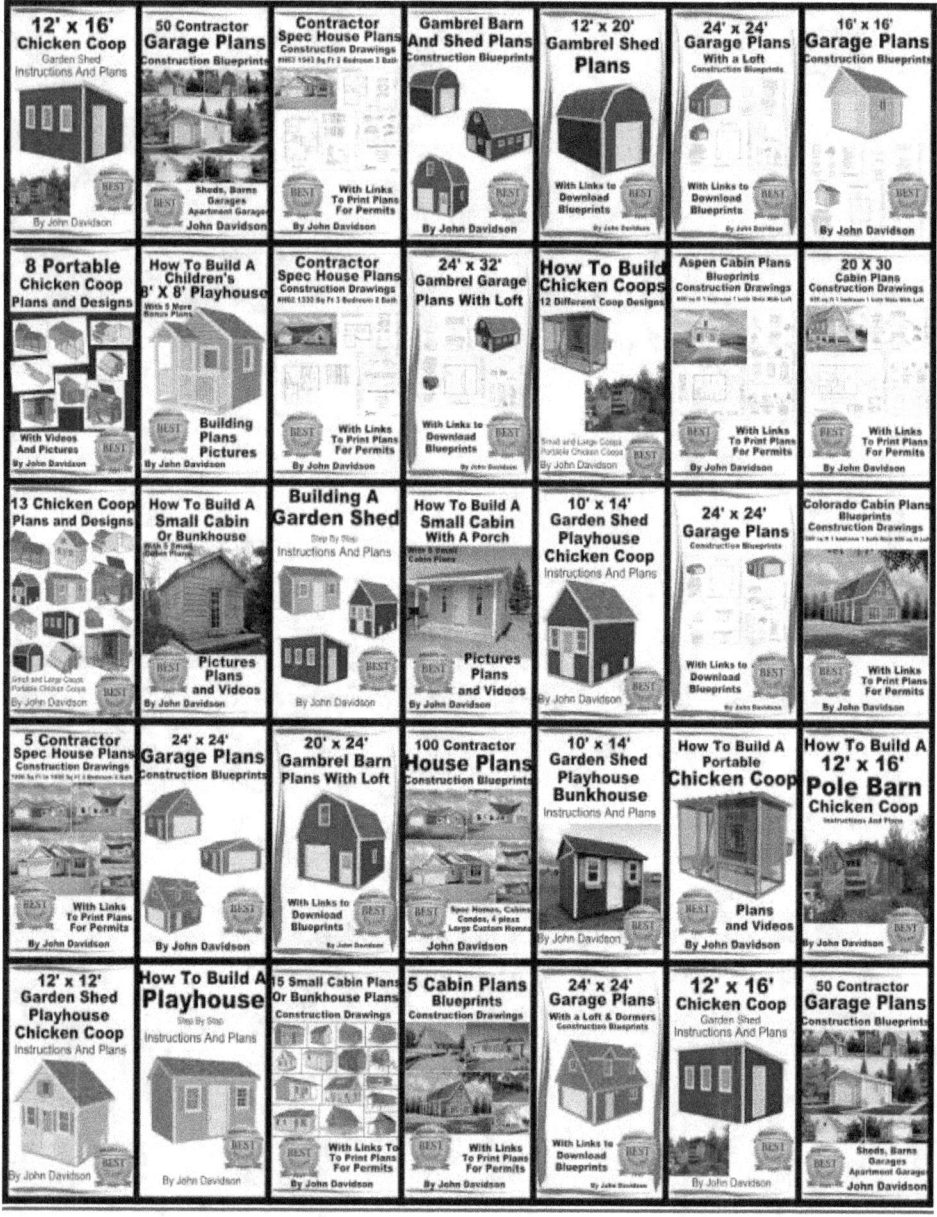

Entrepreneur Book Series

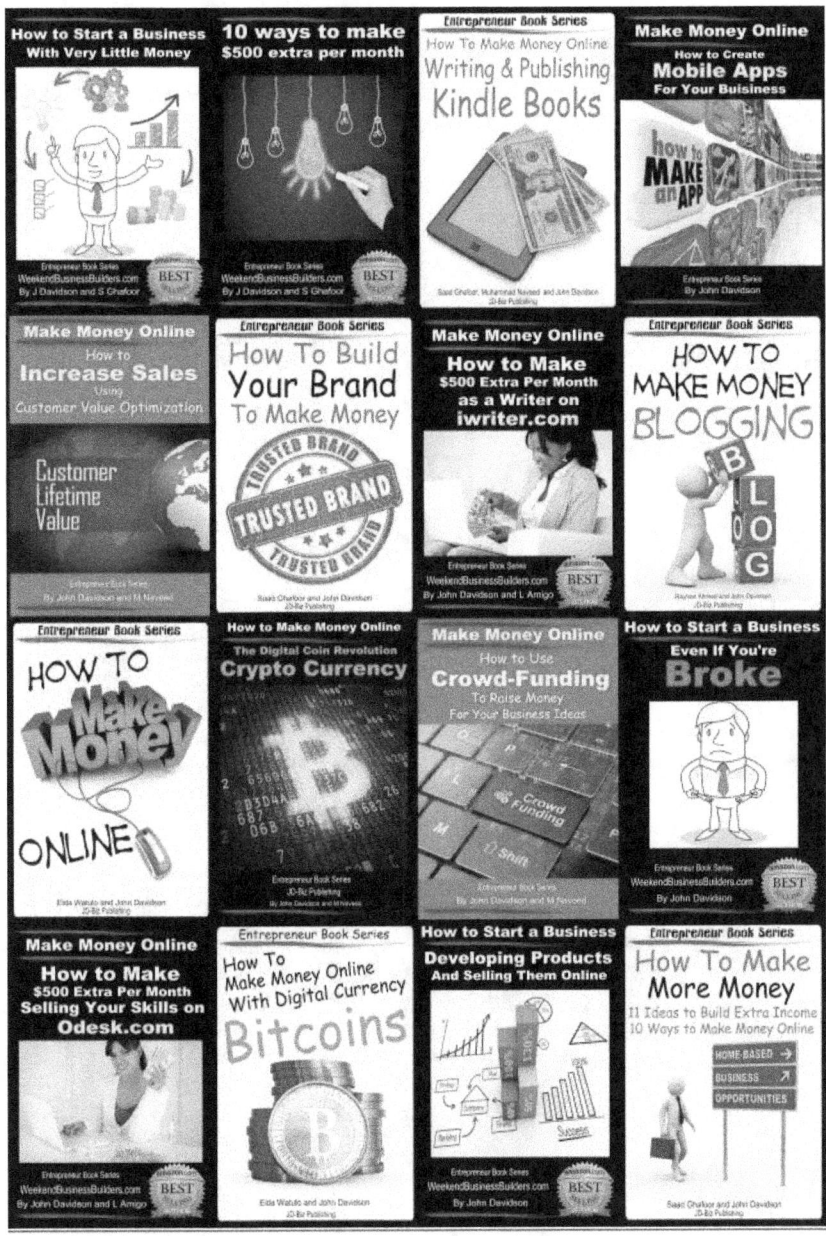

Our books are available at

1. Amazon.com

2. Barnes and Noble

3. Itunes

4. Kobo

5. Smashwords

6. Google Play Books

Publisher

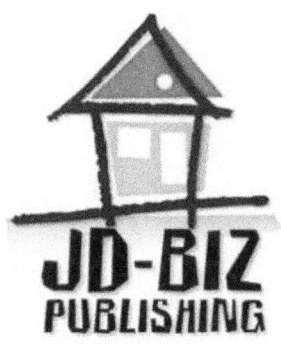

JD-Biz Corp

P O Box 374

Mendon, Utah 84325

http://www.jd-biz.com/

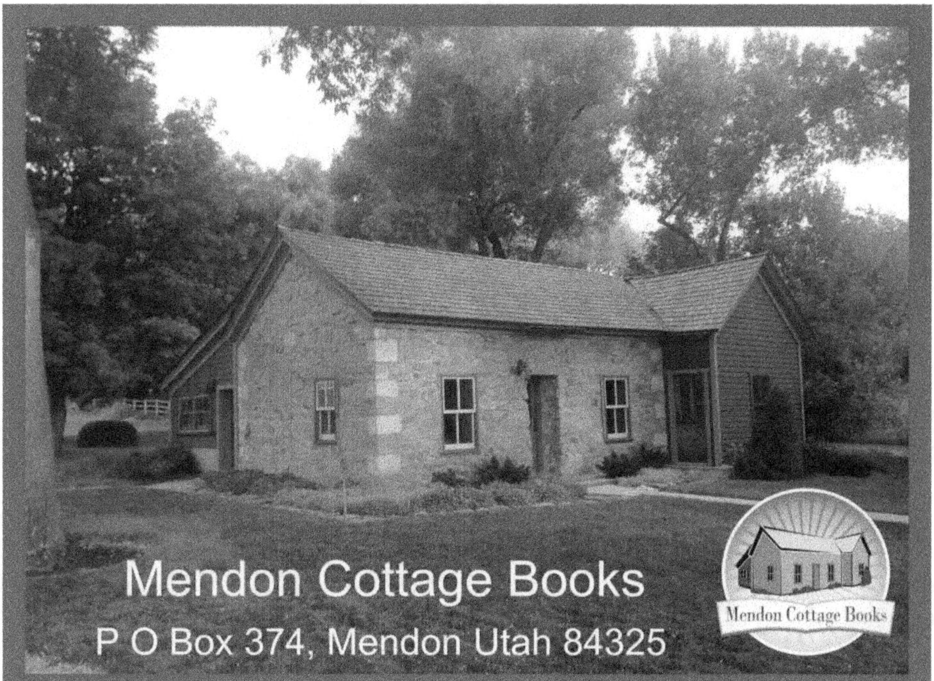

Mendon Cottage Books

P O Box 374, Mendon Utah 84325

www.ingramcontent.com/pod-product-compliance
Lightning Source LLC
Chambersburg PA
CBHW070511290526
45790CB00003B/1192